The Girl in the Mirror

Finding Freedom From the Image We Expect of Ourselves,
and Loving Who We Were Created To Be

By:

Pamela Martin

DEDICATION

This book would not be in your hands today if it were not for the love of my family and friends who believed in me when I did not believe in myself.

My husband Jeff and my parents, Jim and Fran Dixon have always encouraged me, and if not for their support I would not be who I am today. Without the unconditional love of my children, Paul and his wife Kaylah, Samuel and his wife Lindsey and my grandchildren, Elias and Jubilee, I would never have made it through some of my darkest days.

My friends Christy St. Pierre and Kelsey Byers, who stood beside me and lifted me up when I couldn't stand on my own and Stephanie Paasch, who encouraged me to finish this book when I thought I could not, you have my undying gratitude and love.

To my Lord and Savior, Jesus Christ. When at my worst, He loved me still. Without Him there would be no Hope.

*This book is dedicated to my grandchildren,
Elias and Jubilee with much love.*

INTRODUCTION

Everyone starts somewhere. I began my journey almost 50 years ago and it has been an interesting ride. I decided I wanted to share my story after talking with so many women who felt hopeless when it came to achieving lasting weight loss and finally feeling good about who they are. Unfortunately, in this society women often tie their worth to their weight. I fell into this trap at an early age and it took years for me to claw my way out. My hope with this book is to shine the light and help women see they are so much more than their weight on a scale.

Weight loss, when achieved for vanity's sake is never satisfying, nor is it ever long lasting. The fact remains that we age and as we get older, we change. If we are setting our sights on a number on the scale to determine our worth, we will always be chasing that number and we will always be failing. Weight loss must come from a healthy mindset. The reason must be so much deeper than our outward appearance if we want lasting results. It is then that it becomes life changing and it was only when I discovered this secret that I was set free. Gaining a healthier mindset and learning how to be more disciplined was something that would serve me in a much greater way in the years to come as I was faced with tragedy. Having these things in place was instrumental in maintaining my health in the most difficult chapter of my life.

My journey is not over, but I now have a clear path to run on and I know how to get where I want to go. I hope this book will help others find their freedom and see the beauty that they possess no matter what their weight may be.

CHAPTER 1 - FARM GIRL

"After years of telling myself I was overweight and that I was not good enough, I created what my mind believed."

I want to start out by saying that I did not begin my life with a weight problem. I wasn't born overweight. I wasn't an overweight child or teenager either, but after years of telling myself I was overweight and that I was not good enough, I created what my mind believed. Growing up on a farm I had a very happy childhood. My parents were both home with my brother and me every day and life was slow and easy as a child. I was very active and spent most of my days following my dad around the farm. I even had a pony. Ironically, her name was Sugar. I bottle fed baby pigs and calves, raked hay for my dad, and threw the hay out of the back of a pickup truck. I was a natural nurturer and would spend hours cuddling our puppies in the barn because I didn't want them to cry. We were in the local 4-H club, so our summer was very busy getting our livestock ready for the county fair. I did not spend hours and hours in front of the television. I spent them in the sunshine, living the farm girl life.

Like most farm families, mealtime was a big deal. Breakfast was the full country breakfast of eggs, bacon, and my mom's delicious homemade biscuits and gravy with homemade jelly. A nice lunch of bologna sandwiches on soft white bread and mayonnaise with dessert to follow. Later in the evening, my mom would cook an amazing supper consisting of fried foods and mashed potatoes with more dessert. This was the norm for me growing up. This is just the way we cooked and the way we ate as a family. Farm families work hard, and my dad was always in amazing shape. Even now, at the age of 75, he still bales hay, works cattle and rides horses like he did 50 years ago.

My love of food started early, and as I grew and matured, like most girls, I developed a very unhealthy relationship with food.

Growing up in the 70's and 80's it was the time of dieting. Fad diets were everywhere and the lower the calories the better. Diet soda was new and artificial sweeteners hit the market. Being thin was in and if you had a girlish figure, you were considered overweight. I fell into that last category of course.

In high school I very easily fell into binge eating. At the time I didn't know what that was but looking back I can see it so clearly. I always skipped breakfast, and my lunch consisted of nothing but two slices of bread from my lunch tray. When I got home from school at 3:30, I would devour a package of cookies before supper. Yes, a complete package of cookies. I did this all through high school and all the while saw myself as overweight, when in fact I was not. I wasn't very healthy, but I was not overweight, not even close, but the image I saw in my mind was not the image in the mirror. Actually, the image that I saw in the mirror was not even accurate. I would point out every inch of my body that was flawed. I was constantly telling myself how awful I looked. My body image was so distorted that no one could convince me otherwise. This set the stage for years of yo-yo dieting and feeling like a failure when they didn't work. The more I failed, the worse I felt about myself. My idea of eating healthy meant super low calorie and my idea of a healthy weight was stick thin, which I could never achieve. This low self-esteem seeped into every aspect of my life. I was so self-conscious and never felt good enough, smart enough or pretty enough. I hid my insecurity very well. Although I was quiet, I always had a lot of friends. My high school years were great, but behind the smile was an insecure girl who felt inferior to her peers.

I played the comparison game, and in my mind, I always came up short. It is exhausting and painful when you play that game. Every day I would look at other girls and judge myself against them and no matter what, I was never as pretty, as skinny or as smart as they were. I was quiet and somewhat shy, so I hid so much talent in my younger years. I can remember feeling so defeated when I would almost win the contest, or almost get the best grade but didn't and it was because I did not let my talent shine, too afraid of what someone would say to me. Too afraid that I would be judged as harshly as I judged myself.

By the time I was 25 my self-esteem was rock bottom and so was my metabolism. I was married and had two, healthy little boys by that time, yet reading my journals from that period of my life I can see that I was consumed by my weight. In the middle of writing about something wonderful one of my sons had done, I would interject something about my weight and how if I could only lose 10 pounds how happy I would be. I cringe as I read those entries now. I see a young, beautiful girl with so much going for her blinded by the world's idea of beauty and happiness. I was not overweight at that time. In fact, I was at an ideal weight, but in my mind I always had 10 more pounds to lose then my life would be perfect. This set off alarms in my mind that would inevitably lead to my binging which would then lead to my feeling horrible about myself. A never-ending cycle would eventually lead to a real weight issue in later years.

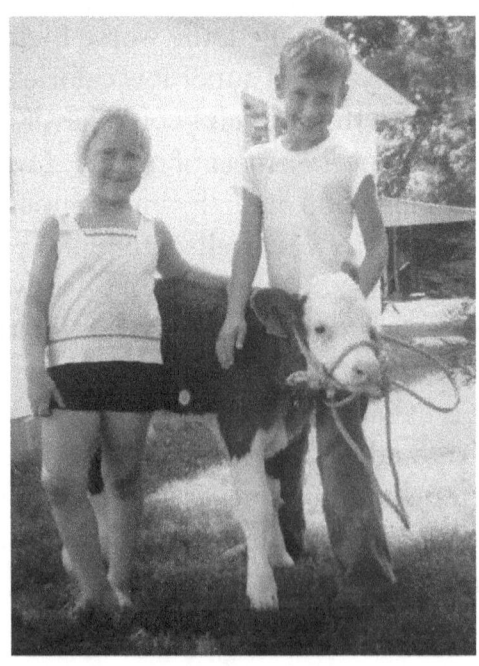

Chapter 2 – THE GIRL IN THE MIRROR

"If I had only seen the girl I was and the girl everyone else saw, and not the girl I perceived I was looking at in the mirror."

When I say I tried every diet out there, I am not kidding. Some of the many diets I tried involved eating nothing but yogurt. I would eat yogurt morning, noon, and night then walk my legs off for exercise. I ate nothing but fish sticks and green beans at one time and would sometimes splurge and have applesauce. I cannot even count the times I joined a very popular weight loss group. I would religiously go to weekly meetings, starving myself all day so I'd see a drop on the scale, sit through a pep talk, then stop by Dairy Queen on the way home because I 'deserved it'. I sent off for diets I found in magazines, I ate nothing but salads, I even had laser treatments that were supposed to be like acupuncture and affect my appetite. Then there was the period of time when all I would eat was cereal. I felt terrible but had no idea why. I didn't know then that nutrition affects not only the body but also mood.

I wasn't quite so positive back then and I believe it all goes back to my poor nutrition. I would lose weight, but it would return with a few extra pounds, or five. This went on all through my 20's and 30's. I was on an endless cycle of calorie restriction, food group restriction and binge eating. The diet wagon was going full speed ahead and every time I would fall off I would run to catch it and jump right back on again, this time with a new strategy to gain control. I truly felt if I wasn't on a diet, I was doomed. Looking back at these years as I write this makes me see how many years I wasted feeling bad about myself. If I had only known then what I know now. If I had only seen the girl I was and the girl everyone else saw, and not the girl I perceived I was looking at in the mirror. I would stand in front of the mirror and pick apart every area of my body. My legs were too big, my nose was too long, and my stomach was never flat enough. I seriously made myself miserable and it was all self-inflicted. I didn't have anyone telling me I wasn't good enough. In fact, my family would tell me I was wrong and I needed to stop saying these things to myself, but I just didn't see what they saw. My view was so twisted and if I could speak to that girl now, I would tell her she is enough. She is beautiful just as she is, and I would tell her to stop comparing herself to the world because the world is not what it seems. Magazine airbrushed models are not reality.

The problem I had was not really about food at all. My problem was internal and so much deeper than just overeating. I have no idea how it came about in my life, but it was deep and it took more than a few years to uncover. Even today, if I am not careful I will find myself thinking those old thoughts. The difference now is I realize what I'm thinking and I make a change immediately. I have so much more confidence now and changing my relationship with food has played an enormous role in that, because once I was successful at losing the weight, I realized I was capable of doing anything I set out to do.

I continued my search for lasting weight loss success and I went to my doctor. I was so desperate by this time, I was willing to do anything to lose weight and gain will power, because I believed I did not possess such a thing called will power. With nothing more than a 5-minute appointment, my health care professional prescribed me a potent drug that would solve all of my weight gain woes. I was so excited to get started. Finally, I would have this monkey off my back and be in charge of my own body. Food had such a hold on me that whether I ate or not I felt guilty. If we went out to eat at a restaurant, I could not enjoy my meal one bit. I would crave it and look forward to it, but as I ate my meal the thoughts would run through my mind that I was gaining weight and I was such a failure. By the time the meal was over, I would be miserable and usually would voice my discontent out loud which would not please anyone I was with. I was out of control and very unhappy.

So, imagine my excitement when my doctor prescribed a drug that would suppress my appetite and was guaranteed to help me lose weight. I ran home and anxiously waited for bedtime when

I would take my pill. In just a few days, I lost 7 pounds. I was floored and thought I was finally free. I was going to lose weight and feel amazing. Then one afternoon a few days in, something went wrong. I remember going into my bedroom and feeling as though I wanted to escape my body. I was panicked and scared and did not know why. My heart was racing and I had this terrified feeling inside. The medication was causing a panic attack and I thought I was going to die right then and there. Needless to say, I never took another pill. It was no surprise when the weight came right back on. By this time, I was in my 40's, 216 pounds and about to give in and just settle with what I thought was my destiny. Something told me there had to be a way. There just had to be some way to lose weight and keep it off. I had never been into exercising properly and had never stepped foot into a gym. Eating clean was a buzzword by this time, and I started looking into what exactly that meant.

    The last effort I made before finding the method that set me free also involved a doctor. This time I went to a holistic doctor because I thought things would be different for some reason. She did very extensive blood work and determined that everything was perfect, but I just could not seem to lose weight. She prescribed what she actually called a miracle medication and she knew I would lose weight, no question about it. It involved injections into my stomach daily, which I did for months and months. I did this, because I wanted to be free from this dieting addiction. I wanted to be free from the negative thoughts and pressure I constantly put upon myself.

    While growing up, my mother would tell me to stop talking down about myself. She was always quick to correct me if I was being negative.

    One of her favorite things to say to me was: "What you say is what you'll be."

    Turns out, she was right. I found that mindset is half the battle. So, daily I would stick a needle near my belly button and inject insulin. I was so desperate to find answers and convinced that medically there had to be a reason my body would not release weight. The one thing all of these doctors had in common, although their prescribed treatment was different, not one physician ever considered changing my nutrition. No one asked what I was eating daily, or how often I had a meal. No one asked why I wanted to lose the weight or made any suggestions towards my food selections. They took out their pad and wrote me a prescription for a pill or an injection and sent me on my merry way, and I took it and did what they told me to do because they were the professionals and knew what to do. Except those things didn't work. The daily injections that were supposed to be the miracle drug, did nothing for me. No weight was lost. Nothing changed and once again, I was frustrated and quickly losing hope.

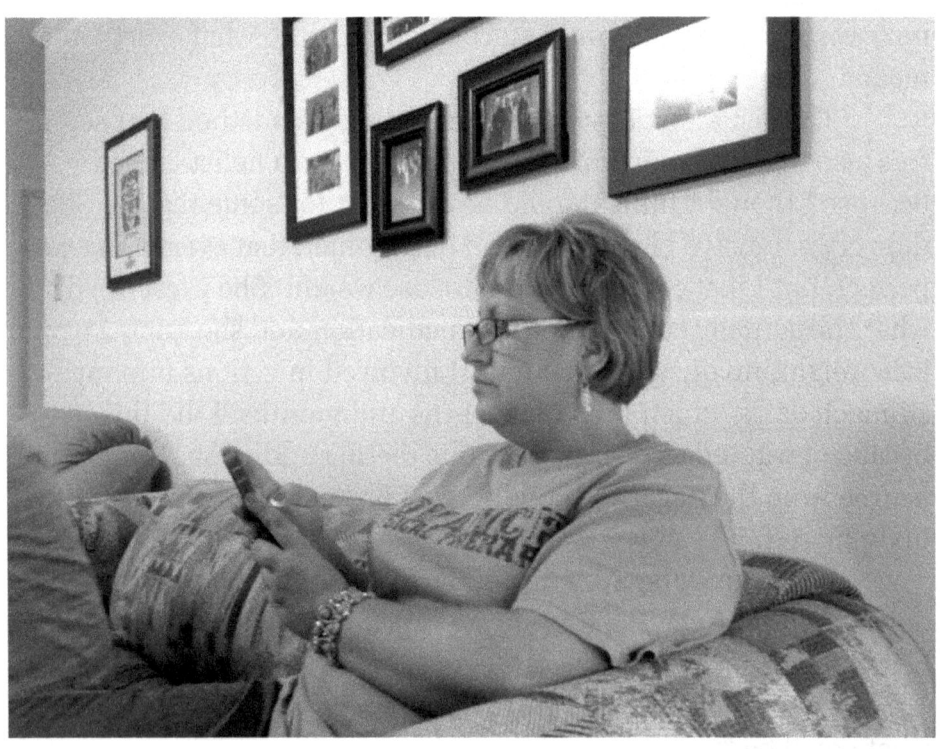

Chapter 3 - STEPPING OUT OF MY BOX

"My reason to make this change far outweighed my fear of being in this place doing things I had never done before. When you reach that point, you truly do become unstoppable."

I don't remember exactly how I got to the point of contacting a health coach. All I remember is feeling completely at rock bottom. I was losing this battle and I was tired. I was more than tired. I was exhausted. Obesity was in my family genetics. Although my mom never had a weight problem, it was still in my genetic makeup, so I just assumed this would be my destiny. I spent so much money through the years on diet after diet, doctor after doctor that I was embarrassed to even suggest that I do this one last thing…but something within me pushed me forward and I made the appointment. I knew nutrition was the answer. I also knew I had no idea what nutrition really meant.

After talking with her I was surprised to find that I needed to eat more than I was eating and more frequently. I wasn't sure I agreed with her about this. This went against everything I had ever heard or done. How can you lose weight and eat every 2 to 3 hours? I was scared to even try that suggestion, but I followed her recommendations and stayed on point and the weight started coming off. Slowly but surely my body started releasing weight for the first time in many years, and I was eating more food on a regular basis then I had ever eaten before and I felt happy on the inside, which was something I had not felt for a very long time.

The next thing I knew I was feeling more energy than I had ever felt before and I hired a personal trainer to take me into the next phase of my journey. This was truly life changing for me and is the catalyst for where I am today as a certified personal trainer. Honestly, if anyone had told me that one day I would be showing people how to fuel their body properly and be a certified trainer, I would have laughed. It was never in my plan or even a thought. It just goes to show that you never know where your journey will lead you if you just follow the path.

When I started my clean eating regime, I weighed 216 pounds. The last time I had weighed that was when I was pregnant with my youngest son. I felt older than I was and certainly looked it. My fitness level was very low. Walking into the gym for the first time was terrifying. Imagine a 45-year-old overweight woman with low self-esteem and poor body image walking into a gym filled with perfect bodies doing exercises she had never seen before. To say I was intimidated is putting it very lightly. The point I want to bring out here is, even though I felt out of place and very uncomfortable, my desire to change was greater than my fear. My reason to make this change far outweighed my fear of being in this place doing things I had never done before. When you reach that point, you truly do become unstoppable.

I remember the first time my trainer asked me to do a box jump. It wasn't actually a box jump like you are probably thinking. It consisted of jumping a foot off the ground onto a step. I could not do it. I would start, but my body would not follow through. I laughed it off, but inside I was dying of embarrassment. How could I not hop up on a step? That is how far I had gone down the path of unhealthy living. I was 45 years old and unable to hop, or even step up very high for that matter and it just spurred me on. I was going to regain what I had lost and I wasn't stopping until I reached my goal.

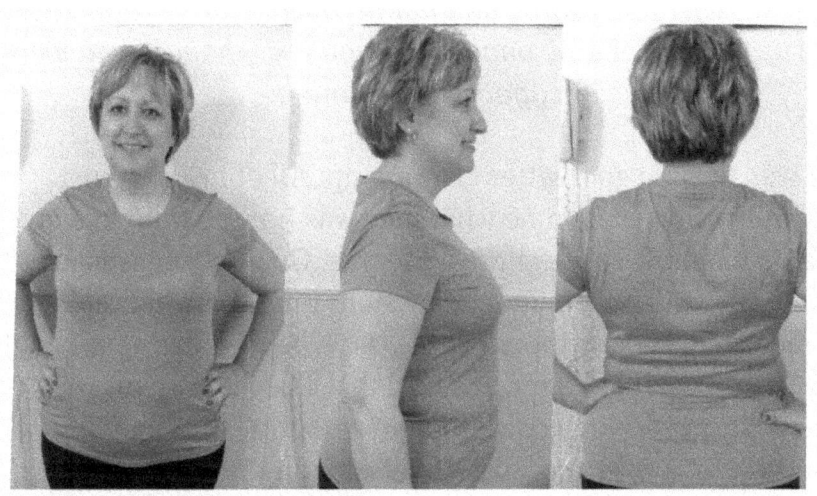
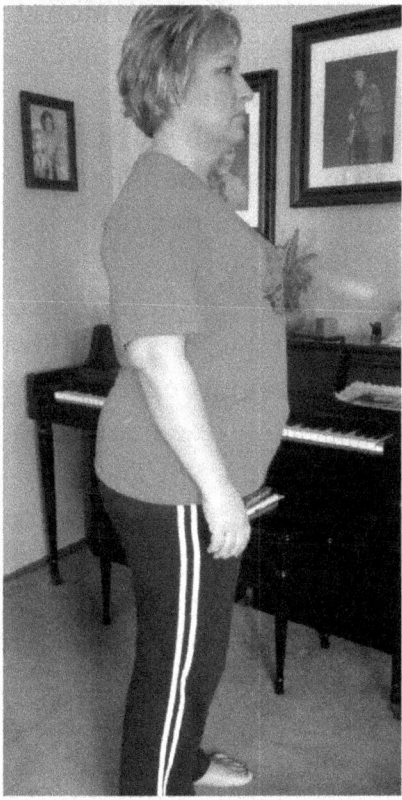
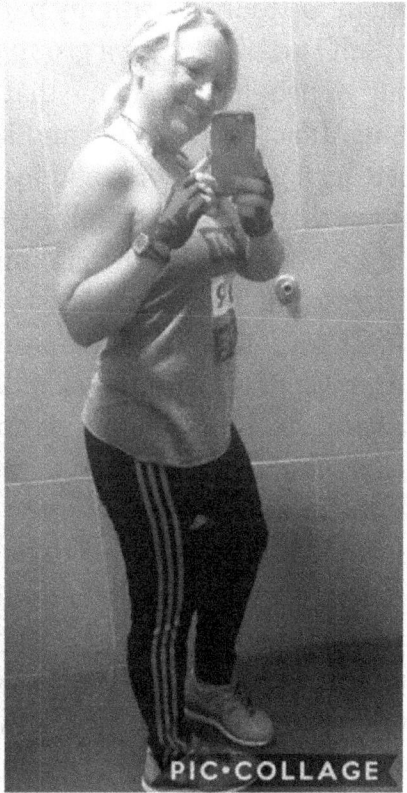

Chapter 4- GOAL SETTING

"When you get this far down you do one of two things; give up and live a life of defeat, unhappy and not in touch with your potential, or rise up and become stronger than you ever thought you were ever capable of becoming."

    I was never a goal setter growing up. All of my life I just rolled with the flow and come what may was how I would live my life. That is just how I thought real life was. Goal setting was just something they talked about on television. It wasn't what real people did. That was my thought at least. When I found that I could actually be successful and reach a goal that I never thought was possible, I started taking goal setting more seriously. I actually, for the first time set a goal and I was determined to reach it. A year after I began my journey with my personal trainer and nutritionist I found myself surrounded by a group of highly motivated people. This group of people showed me that goal setting wasn't just some hokey thing. It actually worked and I saw it work with my friends.

    Setting a goal is more than just wishing for something. It is determining that you are capable of attaining something that will be beneficial for your life. It is disciplining yourself and making yourself accountable instead of just going through life by the seat of your pants. You actually do have a say in how things turn out. If you are not a goal setter currently, I challenge you to start now. Start by setting a small goal, maybe just 30 days out. Make it something that is attainable, but don't be afraid to make it a little scary. The scary goals are the ones that cause massive growth. I like to say, set a goal that you would be embarrassed to tell your mom about, then go tell your mom. When you step that far out of your comfort zone you can't turn around and go back. Once you have spoken your vision to someone, you have set the wheels in motion and you can do nothing but move forward. That is the only way you will ever succeed in breaking out of the box you have put yourself in.

You may ask what made me come to the place where I finally succeeded. Honestly, I had nowhere to go but up. I was rock bottom and I knew I did not want to stay there. When you get this far down you do one of two things; give up and live a life of defeat, unhappy and not in touch with your potential, or rise up and become stronger than you ever thought you were ever capable of becoming. I never knew I was a strong person until I hit the bottom of the so-called barrel. It isn't a great place to be. Imagine the bottom of a barrel if you will. What is down there? Usually stinky, leftover garbage that no one wants to be near. Can you visualize that? How does it make you feel? Probably pretty uncomfortable to just think about, right? Well, that's how I felt and I did not want to stay there. Little did I know how this decision to take control of my life would come to serve me in a much greater way just a few years later.

As I began moving toward my new health, I began learning new ways of thinking about food. I had developed an unhealthy relationship with food. To me, food was the enemy and I was at its mercy. I did not look at food as fuel, but rather entertainment, fun, comfort and a reward. If I was sad, I deserved something from the "bad list". If I was happy, it was time to celebrate with a treat. Every emotion was tied to food and I would use it as my excuse for everything. Then I would overindulge, because I deserved to in my mind, and then the guilt would come. I would beat myself up, telling myself what a failure I was and how I would never be successful if I kept doing what I was doing. I said things to myself I would never speak to another soul. I was such a mean girl to myself and as time went by, I started believing all of those things I spoke to myself. My self-esteem plummeted and the number on the scale went up. What you think about really does affect the outcome of who you become. I was so much more than what I believed I was, if only I knew then what I know now. If only I believed in myself the way I do now. What a difference it would have made in my life and perhaps the lives of those around me.

Luckily, it is never too late and I started getting a healthier outlook on food and on myself. As I became successful I started seeing myself as someone who was worthy of success. I attribute this to nutrition. What we put in our body affects so many aspects of our life. It does so much more for us than just keep us alive. What we put in our body affects our outward appearance, but it also affects our mood and our thoughts. Just like if you give your car watered down fuel, it won't run as smoothly as if you give it premium fuel, your body can't be the miracle it was made to be if you feed it processed food and refined sugars. Studies have been done on the effects of food on our mood and thought process and shows that mental outlook and perceived stress is reduced when a clean diet is implemented. I don't need a scientific study to convince me of this. I have lived it first hand, and honestly, I will never go back to eating the way I did before. The emotional wellness I have experienced far outweighs the taste of any food I could eat. I challenge you to just eat clean for two weeks and see how much better emotionally you feel, not to mention physically. You will not want to go back to the old ways and you will wonder what took you so long to change.

    As my mood changed, my thought process around food also changed, and it was no longer a matter of willpower, or the lack thereof. Cravings no longer controlled me because, my body was now being fueled with what it was craving and I found that I could walk away from the cake. I had grown up thinking I could not succeed because I lacked willpower, which was not the case at all. What I lacked was correct knowledge on how to fuel my body. Processed foods, high fructose corn syrup, refined sugars, all created an addiction and my body craved those things more each time I would eat them. The reason I could not stick to a diet or weight loss plan was because I never stopped feeding my body these ingredients. Diet soda and 100-calorie snack packs of Oreos do not make for a healthy diet. I was still giving my body the inferior fuel and I was running on empty. Once I started putting in the better things such as fresh vegetables, lean protein, complex carbohydrates and lots of water and even healthy fats, I saw a dramatic shift in my body and my mood. I was no longer obsessed with what I was eating and the guilt that used to surround me every time I put food in my mouth left me. For the first time in my life, I could enjoy a meal without feeling deprived or guilty. What freedom that was!

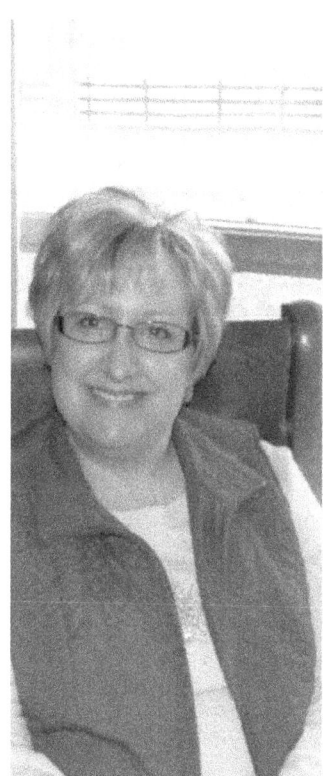
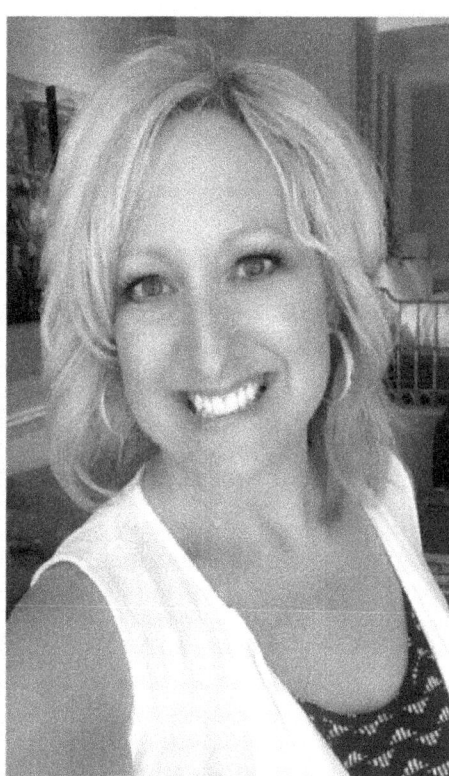

Chapter 5- FITNESS TRAINING

"Every day, we have two choices: we can either choose to stay where we are, or we can choose to do what needs to be done in order to better ourselves."

As my energy returned, my fitness level started improving. I was always active growing up on the farm. You could say I was a Tomboy and loved being outdoors riding my pony and following my dad and brother. I was not, however, a gym rat. In fact, I had never stepped foot in a gym in my entire life until I was 45 years old. As I mentioned in an earlier chapter, I was terrified and it was so far out of my comfort zone. I call the fear of stepping into a gym, "gym-timidated". I never knew what my body was capable of and how remarkable it really is until I pushed it beyond the limits I had set for myself. We are a walking, talking miracle and many of us will go through life never realizing how good we are designed to feel. Putting on lean muscle by strength training gave my body a whole new look. Being one who was consumed by the scale, this did not add up. The number on the scale did not go down quickly, yet my clothing size kept changing. My mind could not wrap itself around this. How I was getting smaller, yet the scale was barely moving was mind-boggling and it was then I realized that the scale was my enemy.

Pushing myself to do something so far out of my comfort zone was evidence of just how determined I had become. I do not naturally do things that make me uncomfortable. Like a lot of people, I like to be comfortable and feel secure. I do not like doing something I am not sure of and I have never liked feeling singled out. So, for me to actually go through with hiring someone to make me workout shows just how far I had fallen and how desperate I was to feel better.

You must make the decision to move forward. You have to want something bad enough to put in the work to get you there. Every day, we make a decision, either it is one of staying where we are or one of change to better ourselves. One way or another, we make a choice. I knew my limitations and I knew I would not ever get the health I desired if I kept doing what I had been doing. I knew enough to know that I didn't know anything about making healthy choices or how to workout to change my body. I swallowed my pride and asked for help. When you are truly ready for change, you will do whatever it takes to get you there. You will find people who have gone before you and succeeded in whatever it is you are working towards. You don't ask advice from someone who isn't where you want to be or who hasn't accomplished what you wish to accomplish. You find the expert, you reach out to people who have been where you are and know how to get you where you want to be. That is the only way you can learn and the only way you will be successful. No one reaches any level of success on their own. Everyone has a mentor or someone they look up to for guidance and the same goes for your health journey. I made the conscious decision to change and went about the necessary steps to learn how to do that.

I very seldom weigh now because it is not an accurate measure of my success. Instead I rely on body circumference measurements, take body fat measurements and the good old, tried and true, skinny jeans test. What the scale does to millions of women all around the globe is set us up for a bad day. If the number doesn't move where we want it to, we beat ourselves up and usually binge eat. If it does show the right number for our mind, it sometimes causes us to overindulge as a reward, at least that is how it worked for me. So, I said bye bye to my scale. I usually weigh-in once a month just to get an idea of where I'm at, but it isn't on my mind like it used to be. I would weigh every day and sometimes go without water or food prior just to see the number I wanted to see pop up. That was not a true measure and it did not serve me well. I encourage you to ditch the scale and start tracking your progress in other ways. If you are in fat loss mode, take body measurements a few times a month. You will feel so much better and you will also see much more progress.

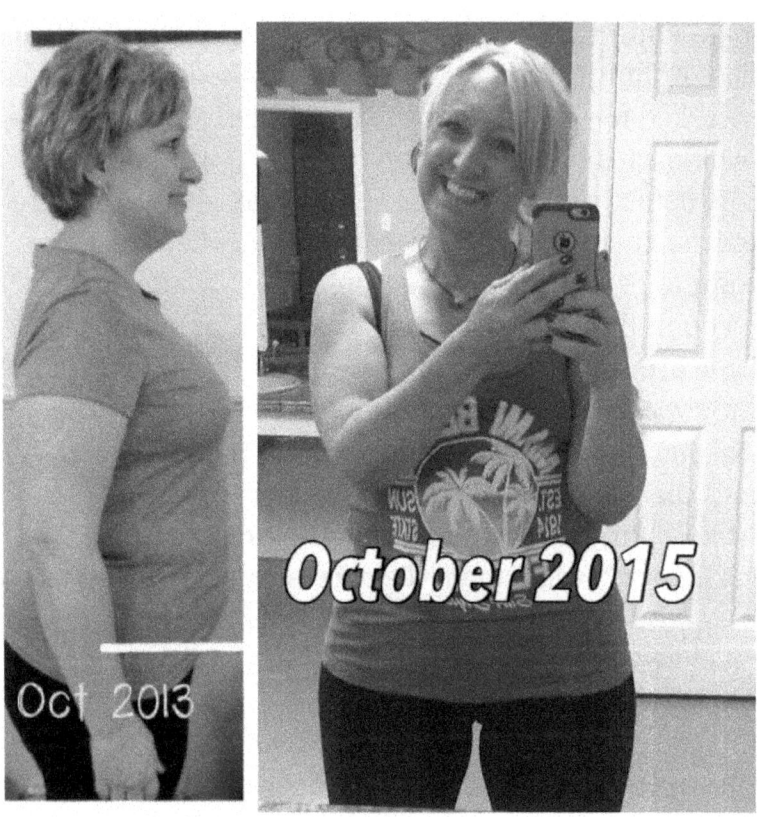

CHAPTER 6- A PASSION IS BORN

"Isn't it amazing how one tiny step in the right direction can lead us to amazing places we never would have been had we not taken that first step?"

      As I continued down my health journey, new things came into my path. I started following a positive, happy woman on Instagram and something about her made me feel better about myself. As I followed her story I found out she used a nutrition line that I had heard of but was skeptical to try. On her recommendation, I took a shot and placed my order for the superfood shakes she used. I was blown away by my results. In just a few days, I started feeling better than I had ever felt before. Clean eating had removed a lot of toxins from my body. What I didn't realize was that our food was deficient in so many minerals and nutrients, so when I started pouring what I was missing into my body on a daily basis, things really took off for me. I had already lost 40 pounds clean eating but I had reached a plateau. I wasn't seeing progress and was frustrated. I lost 6 pounds the first week and was hooked. Not because I broke my plateau but more so because of how great I felt. Knowing it was all natural, without artificial ingredients, made me feel good about what I was putting in my body. Little did I know, but that shake that I purchased because I wanted to break my plateau would lead me to my passion project and an amazing friendship with Kelsey Byers. She has been instrumental in my success, with my fitness and in my business. She has also become one of my most treasured friends.

      I partnered with this amazing nutrition company because it would allow me the vehicle I needed to help others get off the diet roller coaster that I had been riding for all of those years. As I became more involved in the company, I fell in love with the community of other like-minded individuals who were all striving towards the same goal, to help others with clean nutrition. Knowing what it was like to be in bondage to the diet mentality for so long, it felt like my duty to help people know what I now knew. I started telling everyone I knew about this company and without even realizing it, my business was born. Now, not only had I transformed my body and life, I had the opportunity to show others how they could do the same. A passion project had been born. Isn't it amazing how one tiny step in the right direction can lead us to amazing places we never would have been had we not taken that first step? When I started my health journey, it was because I needed to save myself from myself. That step took me to a place where now I can help people worldwide with my global business. Who would have ever thought that little farm girl would be changing lives worldwide?

After 2 ½ years with my nutrition company, I decided I wanted to take yet another step, or leap, out of my box. I started studying to be a certified personal trainer with the National Academy of Sports Medicine. Talk about life changing. I think that shocked me even more than my partnering with a nutrition company. Having only stepped into a gym a few short years prior, I was now on my way to being able to help people on an even larger scale and that excited me, but it certainly wasn't anything I had ever planned on doing. It was just another step on my journey and the door swung wide open for me, so I ran inside before I changed my mind.

Training people in fitness and nutrition has to be the most rewarding thing, outside of raising my two sons, that I have ever done. Knowing I am making a difference in their life by showing them how they can be their very best is something I take very seriously. Not only is your life changed when you gain control of your health, but the life of your family is also affected. Your transformation means everything to the ones who are counting on you. Growing a personal training business alongside my nutrition company is like a dream. It is a huge accomplishment for me because I have gone from poor self-esteem, zero confidence and feeling like I was never good enough, to reaching out and helping other women break free from those same chains. All because I took charge and changed my nutrition. I can't help but wonder what amazing things would happen in the world if more people took their nutrition more seriously and detoxed their body and mind. I don't believe everyone would end up personal trainers, but I do believe good nutrition allows our brain and our body to function at top capacity, puts us in a naturally good mood and makes us much more creative and productive.

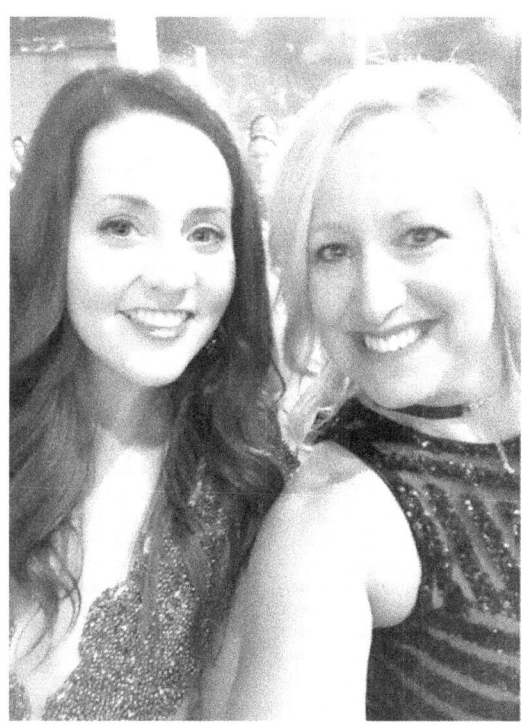

CHAPTER 7- LIFE HAS A WAY OF CHANGING YOU

"When Paul and his wife Kaylah moved back to Missouri, I was so excited and waited patiently for the day Samuel would follow Paul home."

Life has a way of turning the table on you, just when you think you have it all figured out. Life was going pretty great for me at this point in my journey. It was the fall of 2016 and I had joined my business partner Kelsey Byers and several other of my associates in Las Vegas for our company's global conference. I traveled to Las Vegas alone and that was the first time I had really gone that far from home solo. I arrived at The Palazzo excited and left inspired. Our company events are not just motivating, but are also very educational, and I left with a newfound knowledge and a goal that I knew I was capable of reaching. I was ready to get home and fire ahead full-steam, helping as many people as I could reach new heights in their own transformation stories. What I did not know was that in just a few months, everything I was now excited about would be overshadowed by tragedy. I would be faced with the biggest mountain of my life and it would be a true test of willpower, faith, and strength.

    I mentioned in an earlier chapter that I am a mother. I have two sons and my life has always revolved around them. I chose to be a stay-at-home mom because that was all I ever wanted in life. More than anything, I wanted to be a mother and God so blessed me with two amazing, beautiful boys.

    My first son was born on July 11, 1988. I was two years out of high school, which now seems so young, and it was! I was 19 when Paul was born, a kid myself, but so in love with my new baby boy. My second son, Samuel was born on November 12, 1991 and we instantly had a bond. These two boys grew to be the closest brothers I have ever witnessed. I spent my days talking and laughing at their antics. There were countless lazy summer afternoons spent sitting on our porch eating popsicles. Weekly trips to get ice cream at Sonic and deep late-night talks were part of our normal routine. I now look back and see I had an extraordinary relationship with my sons all through their growing years.

When they were in high school, they started a band called *Binding Isaac* with two other friends and they actually allowed me to tag along. As the band mom, I supplied sandwiches and my famous brownies to all the other bands who would be playing with them at the venues. Those were some of the best times I remember. I got to know their friends, and no one seemed to mind that Paul and Sam's mom was hanging around. I certainly didn't mind being allowed to. Our bond was close and strong and to say they were my world would be an understatement. I spent hours praying over my sons. Praying for protection and strength and guidance. I prayed they would make an impact on others and I even prayed for their wives. I had no idea who they would be at that time, but I prayed as though I did. God was faithful. He gave them each a wonderful wife. He guided them and blessed them, and life was amazing for us.

For several years, both of my sons lived in Texas. Paul had moved there to get his Master's degree, which he earned from Southwestern Baptist Theological Seminary. He mastered in Archeology and Biblical Studies. Samuel followed his brother a short time later to start his college career. When Paul and his wife Kaylah moved back to Missouri, I was so excited and waited patiently for the day Samuel would follow Paul home. While we waited for his return, Paul became a daddy. My first grandchild was born on December 15, 2014. Elias James Martin came into this world and with him came new joy and life. People always talk about how wonderful being a grandparent is and I could not imagine just how wonderful until this little smiling cherub came into our lives. My family was evolving and I was ready for the new chapter and adventure that was sure to be on the way.

In August of 2016, that day arrived and Samuel along with

his new wife, Lindsey, moved back to Missouri. We were together again as a family in the same state, only 40 miles apart instead of 700 and I was at peace. I was planning fall adventures to the pumpkin patch, family holidays with everyone around the same table and vacations to beaches and mountains. The fun was just beginning and now that I was also a grandmother to Elias, life was pretty perfect...but, as I mentioned earlier, just when you think life is perfect, it has a way of flipping its switch on you.

On October 10, 2016, I had just arrived at the gym after my job as a secretary at an elementary school when I got a call from my daughter-in-law Kaylah. My oldest son was being taken by ambulance to the nearest hospital. Fortunately, it was in the same town that I was, so I could get there quickly. I rushed as fast as I could to their apartment to get my 10-month-old grandson. We spent the night waiting on tests before traveling to a bigger hospital. Things were not looking good for my Paul. My 28-year-old son had had a stroke...one that had been brought on by a very rare disease called Fibromuscular Dysplasia. None of us, including my son, had any idea that he had this disease. We were grateful that we had found out about it and were ready to make a plan to get him better. The doctors were amazed by his recovery and he was very quickly moved to a rehabilitation center. He had a long road ahead of him, but he was recovering and all of our hopes were high.

A few weeks after his stroke, I was set to go visit him after work and have dinner. I was so excited when I received a picture of him walking and playing a guitar. I could not wait to spend some quality one-on-one time with my son. The next call I got from Kaylah stopped my world. He had just had another stroke and was being rushed again to the hospital. I fell apart right there in my office but gathered my things and rushed out the door. Driving 80 miles-an-hour through afternoon traffic, I made it to his side to find him talking and I thought things would be all right. Maybe it was just a tiny one and wouldn't affect anything? Things like this didn't happen to my family. This wasn't something he should have to deal with. He was only 28 years old. He had a 10-month-old boy and a baby girl soon to be born in February. Life was just beginning for him. This was just a bump in the road. Surely, things would get better.

    Things did not get better. Things went bad. Bad went to worse, and then the unthinkable happened. His surgeon called us together to tell us that this time, Paul would not recover. This time, there had been too much damage and he would not be coming back from it. My world literally stopped turning. I don't remember what was said after that point as my mind refused to accept any more words. All I remember is crying out, "No, no, no! Not my boy!" over and over again. I can honestly say that was the absolute darkest moment of my life. Looking back, it was the second darkest moment of my life. The absolute darkest moment was when I held his hand as he left us. Any dream or desire that had any meaning up until that point no longer existed for me. My son…so brilliant, so loved, with so much to give to the world could not be taken from this world. It was not possible. Yet, it happened. Just days before, as he laid in the emergency room after the second stroke, he told me he was going to make an impact, make a difference in the world when he got better. Why would this happen? HOW could this happen? I will be asking that question for the rest of my life.

For more information about Fibromuscular Dysplasia go to http://www.fmdsa.org/fmd_info/what_is_fmd

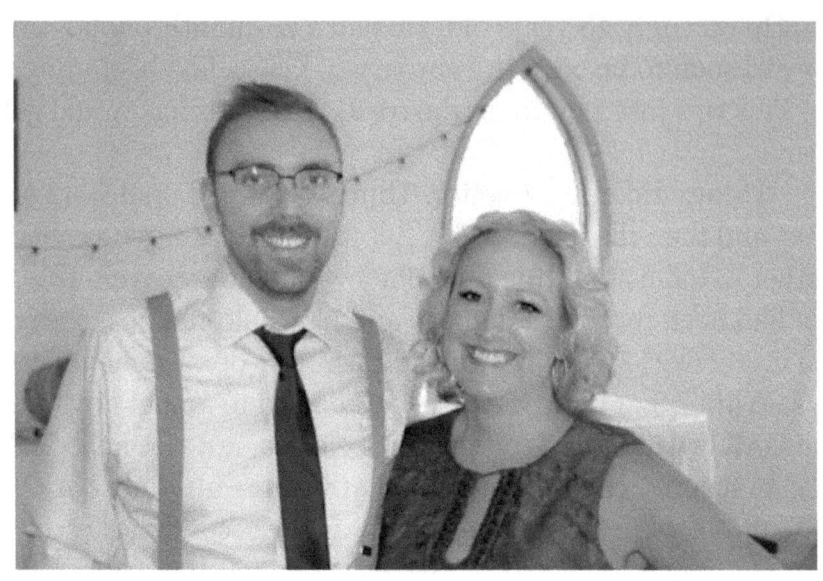

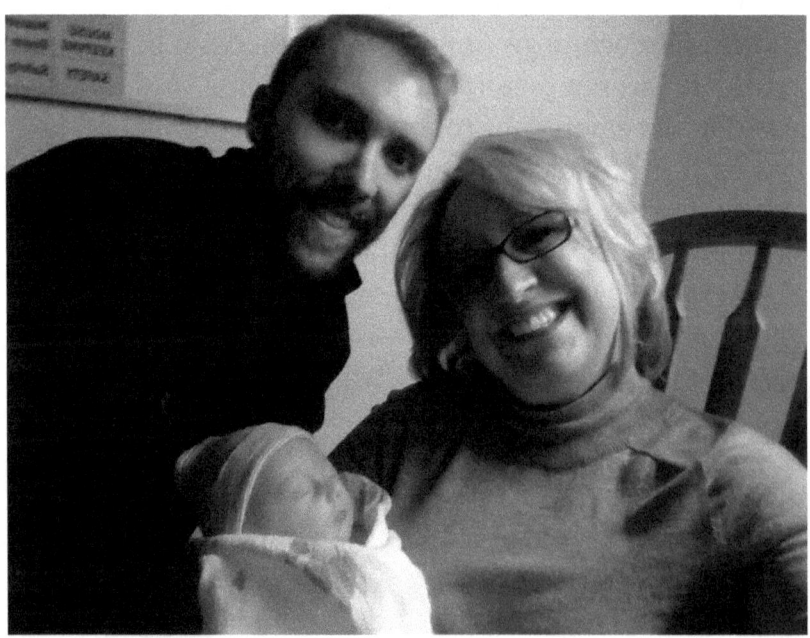

Chapter 8- GRIEF

"On 10/27/16 I held the hand of my boy as he left on his greatest adventure. I will go through this life now with a part of me missing, but the love we had still lives on."

The following is an entry in a blog I wrote to help with my healing. The feelings are raw and painfully real. Writing has always been a private passion of mine. I have always written. I've written in journals. I've written poetry, and I've written short stories. Creating a blog after losing Paul was an outlet for my pain. I never considered it as help for anyone other than myself, but I hope in some way, it will reach someone who is feeling those same feelings and it will let them know they are not alone.

If you can relate to the thoughts I share from my blog or have a friend you think it may help, please share my website, www.amothersstoryofhealing.wordpress.com I would love to help anyone going through grief like this.

Oct. 27, 2016. The day my world crashed. *This has been a day I never considered I'd live. I brought a beautiful baby boy into the world on 7/11/88. I was 19, young I know, but he was what I wanted. A million memories have flooded my mind these last few days and all are just as precious and treasured as the last. I'm still reeling from this turn of events. Not yet comprehending what has taken place. Not yet able to understand. I may never do either of those things. I thought a lot last night about what Paul would say to me. I even asked him how I could do this...how I could let him go. I know Paul would say what he always said to me when he was leaving for one of his grand adventures. "I'll be okay, Mom. I love you. Don't worry."*

I know he's happy and he's rejoicing, and he feels no pain or

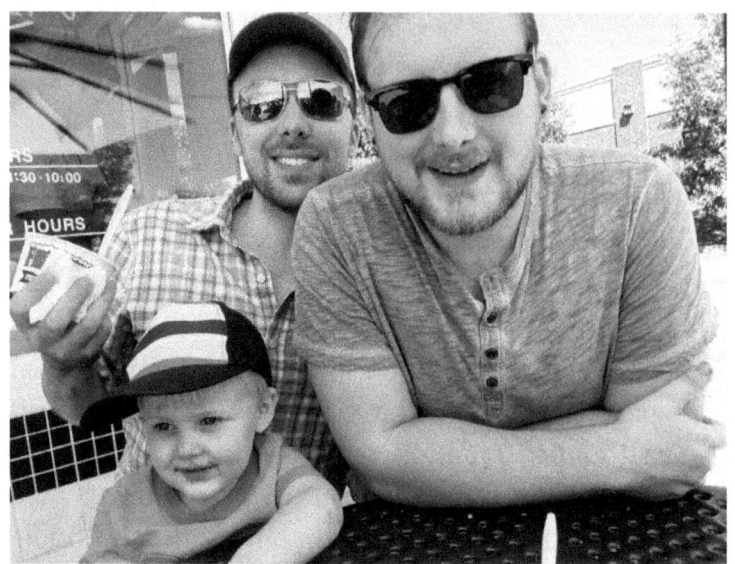

worry. It's those of us who love him who will feel the pain. When he went to college and then on to SWBTS and Cyprus, the only way I could be happy with his choices was knowing he was happy and where he wanted to be. Today, it's no different. Somehow, I will have to accept this and knowing he is happy is the only way I'll be able to.

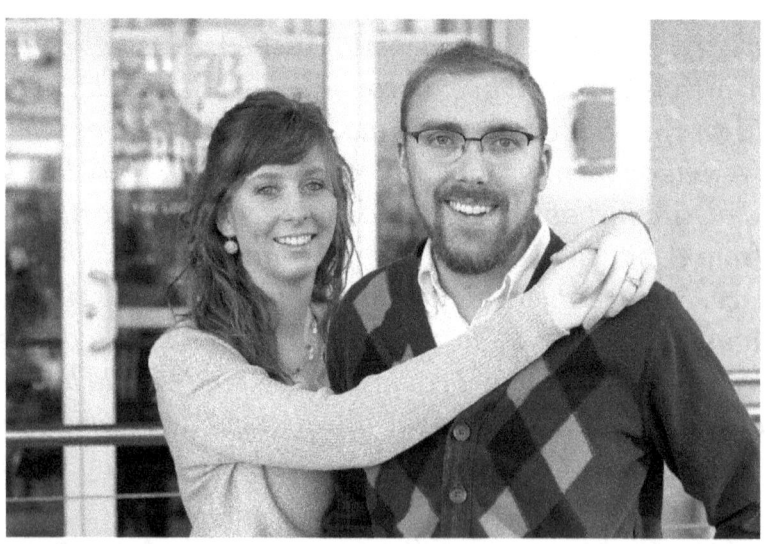

I've been so moved by the posts and messages I've received from those who knew him best. The ones who knew MY Paul, who got to see all of the intricate details of who he was, those who know what I always knew...he truly was a gift. One of a kind. A treasure. I always told him he was my blessing and he always told me he loved me. I will miss him every day until I am reunited with him. The bond we have is not broken. It's strong enough to hold us until he meets me...I know he'll be waiting.

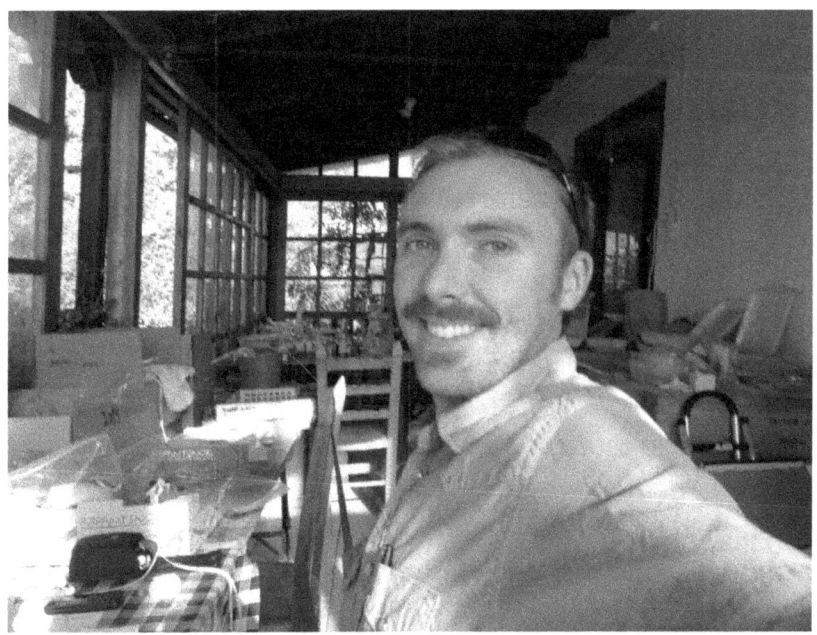

On 10/27/16 I held the hand of my boy as he left on his greatest adventure. I will go through this life now with a part of me missing, but the love we had still lives on. Thank you, Lord, for allowing me to be his mother. I have been richly blessed. I love you Paul Jeffrey Martin.

Chapter 9- NO TIME TO MOURN

"Being strong doesn't mean you can't let go and just fall apart some days. I'm learning that it's needed if there's to be any sort of healing, which at this point, I'm not sure what that looks like. I'll straighten out my crown. I'll even do the wave, but if I don't do it today, that's okay too."

As I went through the days and weeks following my son's passing, I came to know of an awful truth: the world doesn't wait for the brokenhearted. The world must go on and turn and the never-ending clock keeps ticking. For a mother grieving the loss of her son, this was almost my undoing. I had this feeling of guilt that I must regain my focus. I needed to be back to "normal" and go about my day like I had before. I would force myself to go out into public, go to the gym, go get groceries only to find that I was not functioning like I did before. I honestly do not know how I did the things I did for as long as I did. There literally was this feeling put on me by the world around me that my mourning needed to stop.

No time to mourn. This is true, and I never ever thought I'd be on the journey I'm on now. It's the keep it moving part that trips me up. Some days it's exhausting, and I wish I could just stay home and let it all crash around me. Society these days won't allow that. We're expected to keep going...to jump back into mainstream living and act as though nothing has happened to change our world...to be strong but being strong doesn't mean you can't let go and just fall apart some days. I'm learning that it's needed if there's to be any sort of healing, which at this point I'm not sure what that looks like. I'll straighten out my crown, I'll even do the wave, but if I don't today that's ok too.

Something else I felt myself dealing with was my lack of focus. Things that I once found important had gone to the sidelines and my fitness training was one of them. Still, I had that pull to get

in my workouts, to move my body and look as though things were as they once were. I struggled and remember thinking, **I cannot let death win. I cannot allow death to take me too.**

I remember the very first time I returned to the gym a few weeks after losing Paul. I felt like I was just going through the motions, not really focused or feeling into my game. As I did my cardio I looked out over the gym at all the people. Everyone was busy and moving and I thought to myself, *I wonder if anyone can tell I have just lost my son? I wonder if anyone else here is going through what I am going through right now? Do they have any idea of the hurting that is around them at this moment?*
What used to be a daily thing for me was slipping into a few times a week. At first, I felt guilty that I couldn't regain that focus but then I allowed myself some grace.

The one thing I never stopped or fell out of focus on was my nutrition. I had already set the habit of healthy eating, and while I did allow myself more indulgences than before, for the most part I had a plan in place and I stayed with that. I am so thankful that I had the supplements I had grown to love because there were days when that is all I had the energy to make for myself. I truly believe that because I had learned to fuel my body with the right nutrition I was able to deal with so much more than I would have otherwise. My mind was in a positive place and even though I had very many days of darkness and utter loneliness, I never felt myself slipping into the old me or my old habits. I just lost focus on making progress. I was in survival mode and my goal was to maintain some sort of balance until I was through the fog, if that day ever came.

One morning after I arrived at my job, everything came crashing down. The stress of getting back into my old routine of going to work, pasting on a smile and pushing my reality to the back of my mind had reached the end. I went to my best friend's classroom because she was the only person I knew who would listen with a loving heart and literally came undone right there. I had held in my grief so I could carry on my life, go to work and pay the bills but inside, I was literally falling apart.

> *I learned early after losing Paul that the world doesn't stop for the grieving. Life continues on at the crazy pace it travels and most people have to jump back on board regardless of how we feel. Jobs don't allow us to take the needed time off to heal. Bills need to be paid and people need to be fed and onward we are expected to go. I was in a great deal of fog and pain when I had to return to my job. I like to think I hid it well, but it eventually got the best of me and I broke down one morning. It is not normal, or possible to go back to life as usual after losing a child. Especially just weeks after the horrid event. Yet, I had to and I swore I would never be in the position again. I now work from home doing something I am passionate about. I like to think Paul would be so proud of that for me.*

> *Another thing I learned is that people don't like to talk about your grief. You find you are going through this alone, no matter who is around you. Most people in today's society are uncomfortable with sadness and reality of death. Understandably, they don't know what to say, so regretfully, they say nothing. Family and friends tend to avoid the subject, when in reality some days, all you want to do is talk about the one you love. Relive their life. Cry and laugh and not feel like you are making someone uncomfortable by your emotion. I am not asking for pity or sympathy here. Just stating what I have observed in my journey.*

> *One thing I have learned from this is how to comfort the*

grieving. Sure, sending food or flowers is so important the week or two following the event. It is the weeks, months and years that follow that find the family alone and dealing

with the pain. I have just a handful of friends who have stayed the course with me. I can actually count them on one hand, and that's ok. I don't say this to shame anyone. I have not been that friend in the past myself. I think we all, as a society need to learn to care more sincerely and not be afraid of pain and sadness, but to walk alongside someone when they are experiencing it. We all will go through it at one point in our lives. Sometimes, when it is your child you are grieving for, it is more difficult for others to know what to say or do. That is a loss that no one can fathom because it goes against the way things are supposed to work. Yet, it happens, and those parents need so much patience and understanding and care. My son, my first born baby boy. The child I prayed for and made me what I always wanted to be most, a mom, is gone...there isn't anything anyone can say that will make it better, but a hug does wonders. Simple as that.

I have been reliving last October and trying my best to avoid it. That day is coming, and I will have to look it in the face. I want you to know about my son. Paul was an amazing person. He was a joy as he grew from infant to child, to teenager to father. He and I shared a bond and love that will never be broken. I was 19 years old when he was born. All I wanted was to be a mom and he made that my reality. Paul was witty and brilliant. He was creative and as a child always inquisitive about the world around him. We learned together and as he grew I prayed over him to become a fierce and mighty man of God. To be strong and caring. I prayed he would impact others. God was faithful.

Paul was a gifted musician and I truly mean that. He could play anything he wanted to and wrote countless songs. He

loved to write and has over 40 journals that his babies will have to treasure forever. He had a sense of humor all his own and truly loved life. He loved people and he was the best of friends anyone could want. He always greeted me with a hug and when he would leave, another hug and an "I love you, mom". As a teenager he allowed his mom to go with him when he and his band would play and was never embarrassed by the fact that his mom was his biggest fan. He found solace in the woods and would go out to the farm and spend time there, just thinking. He spent a lot of time thinking. He always had a journal with him and a couple of books, just in case a thought came to him he'd want to write down. He had a gorgeous smile and happy eyes and a beautiful laugh. I could go on and on about him. Twenty-eight years was not near enough time with this boy.

So, as I brace myself for the coming days I will openly think of him. I will have days of joy but also sadness and they do go hand in hand. With great love comes great sorrow. It is the price we pay for love, but to avoid sorrow would mean avoiding love, and that would be even more tragic.

I spent a lot of time hiding my pain. I did not want anyone to feel sad, so I would never really express how I was feeling or what I was going through. This was not exactly the best course of action. I really should have sought help, but I think I was trying so hard to make things as they once were, to avoid the reality of my life that I pushed myself to keep going when I really should have just stopped.

It seems I don't really have time to grieve. I've had to go back to work and every day is exhausting. Just to maintain a presentable presence. When all I want to do is stay in my pajamas and drink coffee and cry. If I could just do that until all my tears are gone, maybe I'd be more myself. I have to spend the week in denial, otherwise I wouldn't be able to be in the workplace or in public. When the weekend comes it all falls down and I spend it being faced with reality.

They say it takes time. But really, how much time? I don't think a mother ever gets over losing her child. I was the one who felt his first movement. I was the one who loved him first. I was the one who held his little hand first. It may get softer with time. I hope it does anyway. This pain is unlike any other and I can't imagine feeling this for the rest of my life, but I'll always love him and I'll always miss him so I imagine I'll always feel this pain.

Another day goes by without you.

The lesson I learned and wish others to take away from this is be patient with the grieving. We have no idea how to process our feeling and our mind is being pulled in a thousand directions. Don't ask how you can help the hurting, just observe what they need and step in and do it. During this time someone offering to pick up my groceries would have been a huge help because thinking about what I needed and going to the store to get it was really pushing it some days. It is a time when little things do mean a lot.

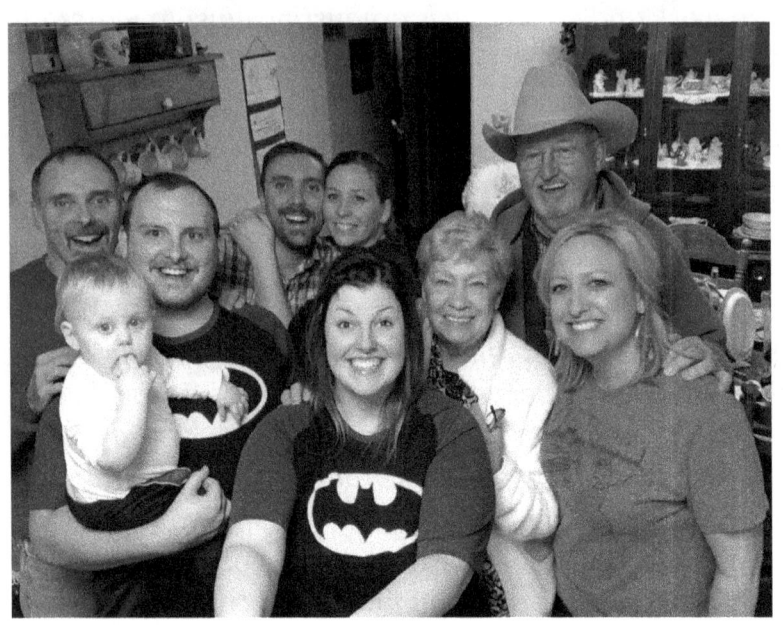

Chapter 10- LEARNING THROUGH SORROW

"I had a confidence I had never had before. I also had a huge reason to push past the fear."

As I write this, it has only been a year and a half since I lost my son. I am far from arriving at a place of joy, but I can see what I have learned through the past year. It is interesting to look back at one's life and see how things have fallen together after falling apart. Losing my son has by far been the darkest hour for me and through that darkness, I have learned many valuable lessons.

After leaving my job, I was able to focus on healing and for the first time, I felt at rest. I didn't have to rush out the door and if I chose to stay in my pajamas all day, I did and I did not allow myself to feel bad for doing so. I knew I needed to find myself again, whatever and whoever that was. I dove into my nutrition business and through that, found that helping others in turn, helped me. Doing something that allowed other people to see that they could be successful and could feel incredible made me feel the same way. This time to myself is when I came to the realization that becoming a certified personal trainer was something I wanted to do and for the first time in my life, I had the confidence to try. The little farm girl I once knew would never have ventured so far out of the box, but pain and loss had taught me the value and brevity of life and if I was to ever do or be what I wanted to be, I had to do something I had never done. I also knew that it would give me more knowledge to help those who were looking to change their health. Now I could show them how to get on track with their nutrition and fitness, setting them up for success.

I also learned that time is the most valuable thing we have. It is irreplaceable and I was determined to never lose another moment with those I cared about most. I was determined to never feel trapped or allow someone else to dictate where I spent my time or what was important. I had a confidence I had never had before and also a huge reason to push past the fear. Once you get in touch with why you want to accomplish something, there really is nothing that can get in your way. One door after another opened for me. Each door scarier than the last, but on the other side of fear was freedom and success and it moved me one step closer to my ultimate goal. Slowly my focus started to return and this time I was more determined than ever, not just to be fit and healthy, but to be who I was meant to be.

Paul led an amazing life. He saw and did so many things, yet he had so much more to do. He wanted to impact the world and use what had happened to him to help others. I wasn't sure how I could do that, but I knew I had to use my own journey. My journey that started out sounding like a weight loss journey but really was so much more than that. It is a journey to finding out what I am truly all about. A journey to free the girl inside who, for so long, counted herself unworthy of the dreams that had been placed within her.

I do have great joy. Even in my sorrow, I can smile. Grief is a strange thing and I don't pretend to understand it. If you think that in losing your loved one you aren't allowed joy, you are wrong. I hope you can still find joy in your life. Yes, it may be different and not the same as before, but it's there. Of course, it's always bittersweet. Where joy used to be complete sweetness, like the best chocolate in the world, now after losing Paul, joy is always bittersweet. Family gatherings where laughter and fun surrounds me always leaves me with thoughts of how much Paul would be enjoying this too. Seeing Elias and Jubilee doing funny things brings joy to my heart, but always makes me think of all he is missing. You see, every joy is sprinkled with the 'what if' or the 'I wish' or 'if only'. I realize this will follow me and all of my family all through our lives now, but that is okay. I'll take the bittersweet because that is what you get when you've loved and have been loved with no regrets and no boundaries.

I still have so many questions and my heart on some days gets so angry at this tragedy. I realize some may judge me for admitting that, but I would venture to say that those who do haven't lost what I have lost, so I give them grace. I know I will find peace and I know God is beside me through all of this and He understands my anger and my questions. So, I will enjoy the silence today and welcome the memories to flood my heart. Tears will come, but I am not afraid of tears. Tears cleanse the soul.

Allowing myself to rest and just grieve was the most important thing I did at this time. There were times when I would find myself feeling guilty for smiling or laughing. Then I realized that to grieve does not mean we lose our joy. If we lose our joy, we have truly lost and I know my joy was everlasting. My faith taught me to trust and to find our joy in the Lord. During those days, my faith felt weak but as I have mentioned before, God has been so very patient with me. He knows my pain and never left my side, even in the darkness.

Chapter 11- I DREAM OF YOU

"My dream ended with us embracing and crying together. It felt like love and it felt like we both knew what had happened, yet we were together saying good-bye."

In this chapter, I am sharing a very personal revelation I had during one of my journal blogs. This particular blog entry recaps my dreams about my Paul.

I am not one that usually puts much stock in dreams. Actually, I rarely remember them, but the other night I had a dream so vivid I don't think I'll ever forget it. It was of Paul.

Like most dreams, a lot didn't make sense. I don't know where we were or what exactly we were doing. What I remember most is the feeling. He was there, wearing a shirt I saw him wear so many times and we were smiling and laughing like we always did. Paul had the most genuine and radiant smile! He smiled with his eyes and that is the sign of a truly happy person I think. I saw his beautiful face and we talked. His brother, Samuel was also in the dream and I watched as they laughed together like they always did. No one ever really knew what those two were talking about, but they could get into the deepest conversations and then the next minute they would both be laughing. Most of the time at something only the two of them would understand. A brothers bond is truly special and they had the most special bond I've ever seen.

I'm not sure why I had this dream. It could be because the next day was a baby shower for his little Jubilee Mae who is due to arrive in a few short weeks. Paul was so excited for a little girl. When the doctor announced they'd be having a girl, Paul cried tears of joy! He was beside himself with happiness. He would say how he was going to teach her to be a strong woman. She would be smart and strong and not fall into the traps so many girls today fall into. He would make sure of that. What a great daddy to his girl he would have been. Which makes me again wonder why this had to happen. Why? I think I will always ask that question. Why someone who was so special, so loving, so brilliant and compassionate would be taken so early in life. He was a doting husband who left love notes up until the day before his stroke, for his wife. He often would surprise her with flowers or tiny gestures of love, like a guitar pick. Sounds funny to most of us, but it meant something to Paul therefore it meant something to his bride.

My dream ended with us embracing and crying together. It felt like love and it felt like we both knew what had happened, yet we were together saying good-bye. I remember when he was in the ICU and we knew his time was fleeting how I would get as close to his face as I could, just to remember every detail. I did that when he was a baby too. I would rock him and just stare at his perfect little face, trying to capture every detail in my heart. I did the same at the hospital, just to gaze at him and put every tiny detail and memory into my heart where I could go and find it when I needed to feel him again.

This journey is far from overt. I have better days but when I have a bad day, it is far worse than before. I think I can only push out the reality so long until it crashes in on me and I'm forced to once again acknowledge the painful truth that I've lost my boy. I'll never understand why. I'll never be the same. I will, however, keep going and I will do my best to teach his precious prince and princess the things I know he wanted them to know. To be compassionate and make a difference in the world, just as he has done.

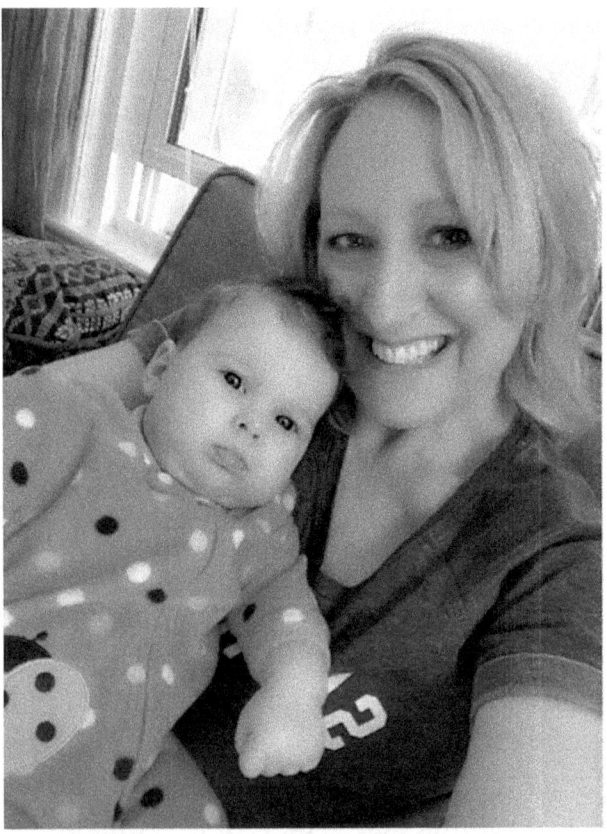

Jubilee Mae blessed our lives on February 2, 2017

Chapter 12- RENEWAL AND BLESSINGS

"What you learn along the way is meant to be passed on. It is also meant to help you through the next storm you will face."

Paul left us two beautiful blessings: Elias and Jubilee. They have been a light during this dark journey. God knew we would need their little faces and sweet kisses to pull us through some difficult days ahead. Having two grandchildren has become my driving force to stay focused on my health and fitness. I have even more reasons to continue on this path I set out on five years ago. When I started this health journey, it was for myself. I did it for me and no one else, but now it has become something I must do for others. My health is important, but so is yours. People depend on you in so many ways. People care about you and if there is anything you can do to be at your very best, it is absolutely necessary to do it.

The last few weeks have been a roller coaster of emotions for me. On February 2 at 3:58 pm, we welcomed Paul's little girl into the world. Little Jubilee. As I stood outside the door and waited for the tiny cry of this little one that would signal her birth, I had the overwhelming feeling that Paul was there. It washed over me in a way I cannot explain but the tears came and I was in a whirlwind. I've never had happy mixed with sad before. It is a perplexing feeling and one I am not sure I want to feel again, although I am sure I will as these two children grow up without Paul beside them. As I stood in that hospital hallway, it all rushed over me. The memories of Paul's birth, the days of his childhood, his laugh, his bright-eyed smile and his final minutes that I sat holding his hand tightly in mine. All within a heartbeat of seconds and then her cry broke the trance and she was here.

I imagined how he would have felt, seeing his newborn daughter. He was so excited and overjoyed at the announcement that they would be having a girl that I could clearly see his face lit up with that gorgeous smile of his as he would have walked from the room to tell the news of her arrival. I could see him holding her, wrapped tightly in her blanket as he propped a book on his lap and read or perhaps wrote something on his computer. He would have had her with him every minute he could, bundled tightly and so proud of his princess.

He would have told her silly stories to make her giggle, funny stories of a piggy princess and a handsome toad. He would have taught her Greek and Hebrew and she would have been a strong, brilliant girl alongside her brother as they learned on their daddy's lap. She will still be strong and brilliant, but the things Paul would've taught are things none of us can possibly teach her or her brother. This is what makes me cry and angry at the same time. I feel they have been so cheated of the life they could've had if only their daddy had been spared. If only the prayers we prayed had been answered the way we wanted them to be. I know, God has a plan, I just wish it included Paul raising his children. I don't mean to sound bitter. I am a healing mother after all. I trust that in time I'll come to terms with all of this, but for now all I can do is wonder why.

The birth of Jubilee has been healing for us even through all of the pain of knowing what she and Paul are missing of each other. She is a delight. A peaceful and content soul, much like her daddy. I feel he is with her as she dreams and will always be there, looking over her and Elias' footsteps through life. Whatever the reason he was taken from our lives I have to trust his children will be ok and will still rise to carry on what their father started. They will make a difference in this world. They will be a change for generations. They will rise up and help others and love unconditionally. Love doesn't die, it is carried on in the hearts of those who have had the privilege to feel it and own it. Elias and Jubilee were loved so deeply by their father that I have no doubt they will always know him in some special way.

Thank you, Paul for the blessing of your little Jubilee Mae and Elias James. They have filled my heart with love and joy. You did good my son.

It is now for Paul's children and the children my son Samuel and Lindsey will one day have, that I continue on my health journey. I see now more than ever before the importance of taking care of the miracle body God has given us. That is what is so important to understand and what you must find on your own journey. You must find out 'why' you want the things you do. Why do you want to lose 50 pounds? Why do you want to work from home? Why do you want to be financially free? Not just the easy reasons, but the REAL reasons. You have to look deep within and be real with yourself. When you do this and you come to terms with your why, you have opened that scary door and you are about to step into success.

My journey is far from over. I have days of sadness and days of joy, but God is with me through them all. I am learning to lean on Him more and allow His peace to comfort me. I will admit, I went through a time of anger and could not and would not understand how or why this happened, but through it all God waited and never left my side. My hope now is that I will take what I have learned from my journey and pass it on to those struggling down this same path.

You may ask yourself how weight issues and grief tie together. My hope with writing these things together is that it will help someone see that life is all about the journey. What you learn along the way is meant to be passed on. It is also meant to help you through the next storm you will face. Looking back, my struggle with my weight and self-esteem never came close to comparing to my struggle through grief and loss. It did, however, allow me to find my voice so that perhaps in some small way, I can make an impact on someone and help them through the muddy valley of their own journey...to help them face the girl in their mirror.

-xoxo

Pamela Martin

NOW IS THE TIME FOR YOUR JOURNEY

I shared 28 wonderful years with Paul. To honor those years, I've created 28 encouraging and supportive journal topics of mindset and health changes to help you get started on your journey to a healthier you.

Goal Planning: The first step is determining what goals you want to achieve. Ask yourself how you want to feel and look a year from today. Set that goal and put a plan in place to achieve it.

Today's Date _____
Accountability Partner _____
Telling someone your goals makes you more 85% more likely to reach them. Tell someone!

List three goals for fitness:
1.
2.
3.

Rate each of the goals on the five principles listed below by placing a checkmark in the appropriate column if the goal conforms to that principle.

Goal	Specific	Measurable	Action Plan	Realistic	Timely

Based on the previous analysis what are potential goal-setting strengths and weaknesses?

Strengths:
_____
_____
_____
_____
_____

Weaknesses:
_____
_____
_____
_____
_____

Below are three opportunities for planning general fitness goals based upon the previous goals discussed. After each one, write two specific, measurable goals that lead to reaching the general goal. In the final space, specify one other general goal and two specific goals to reach it.

1. To improve my _____
    a. _____
    b. _____

2. To improve my _____
    a. _____
    b. _____

3. To improve my _____
    a. _____
    b. _____

4. General Goal: _____
    a. _____
    b. _____

1. Find Your Why

Why do I want to achieve my goals?

Dig deep and peel away the layers of your why statement. If your goal is to lose 50 pounds there is a deeper reason than just seeing that number on a scale or fitting into a certain size. Why? How would achieving that goal change your life? What would it mean to you? How would you feel? Dive deep!

2. Face Your Fear
What is keeping you from starting your health journey? Be honest with yourself and write down all the things that go through your mind that keep you from getting started.

3. Nutrition
How will eating healthy now affect you in the future?

_____
_____
_____
_____
_____
_____
_____
_____
_____
_____
_____
_____
_____

4- Emotional Eater
When you eat because of stress, where does the stress go? What can you do instead of eating to help yourself de-stress?

_____
_____
_____
_____
_____
_____
_____
_____
_____
_____
_____
_____
_____

5. What does your "ideal" body look like?

_____
_____
_____
_____
_____
_____
_____
_____
_____
_____
_____
_____
_____
_____
_____
_____
_____

6. Move Your Body
What fears do you have around joining a gym or working out in general? What steps will you take this week to move past those fears?

_____
_____
_____
_____
_____
_____
_____
_____
_____
_____
_____
_____
_____
_____

7. Healthy Habits

What are you willing to give up and replace with a new, healthier habit?

_____
_____
_____
_____
_____
_____
_____
_____
_____
_____
_____
_____

8. Food Feelings

You have made healthier choices around meals all day. How do you feel physically and emotionally compared to days when you do not make better choices?

_____
_____
_____
_____
_____
_____
_____
_____
_____
_____
_____
_____
_____

9. The Best Part About Me
Make a list of your top ten best character traits.

10. Gratitude

What are you grateful for? Can you think of 10 people or things that you have gratitude for today?

11. Role Models
Who do you look up to and why? How are you on your path to be more like them?

_____
_____
_____
_____
_____
_____
_____
_____
_____
_____
_____
_____
_____

Day 12. I am Proud of Me.
Make a list of 20 things you have accomplished. Think about your life and write down at least 20 accomplishments you have obtained over your lifetime.

_____
_____
_____
_____
_____
_____
_____
_____
_____
_____
_____
_____
_____
_____
_____
_____

13. Visualization

Dive deep and think about where you want to be a year from now. How do you look? What are you wearing? Where are you? How do you feel? See yourself feeling your best, looking your best and being in that place that makes you the happiest. Is it the beach, the mountains, on a special vacation with family? Really spend time visualizing yourself and write down everything. Come back to this place often on your journey and you will find that eventually you will find yourself there in reality.

14. What is Holding You Back?
What are 3 things that have kept you from moving forward in the past? Why do you think you allowed them to hold you back?

15. Plan of Action
How can you push past the things that held you back that you wrote about in #14? Write about 3 ways you can overcome those obstacles today so that you will be successful?

16. Love Yourself

Look at yourself in the mirror. Write down 5 things you love about what you see.

_____
_____
_____
_____
_____
_____
_____
_____
_____

17. I Am...

Write down 20 statements about yourself. Make these power statements of things you are going to achieve, but write them as if they are already reality. (Example- I am at my goal weight of xxx, I am confident and positive, I am building a business that I love...etc)

_____
_____
_____
_____
_____
_____
_____
_____
_____
_____
_____
_____
_____
_____
_____
_____

18. Revisit Your Why

Revisit your Why statement today. Are there more layers you can peel away now that you've been on this self-awareness journey?

19. Today I...
What did you do today that you are the most proud of?

20. Weight Loss Goal

What about losing weight will make my life different?

21. Dear Me,
Write a letter to your 16-year-old self. What would you tell that girl now?

22. What Would You Do?

If you knew you could not fail, what would you do?

_____
_____
_____
_____
_____
_____
_____
_____
_____
_____
_____
_____

23. I Felt Amazing When...

When was a time you truly felt your best? What were you doing then that made the difference?

_____
_____
_____
_____
_____
_____
_____
_____
_____
_____
_____
_____
_____

24. What I Love About Me
Write down 5 qualities you love about yourself.

_____
_____
_____
_____
_____
_____
_____
_____
_____

25. Words I Say
Write down 10 positive words you need to tell yourself today. How are these words different than what you usually tell yourself?

_____
_____
_____
_____
_____
_____
_____
_____
_____
_____
_____
_____
_____
_____
_____
_____

26. Food is Fuel, Not Therapy
What are 10 things you enjoy doing to relax and de=stress that do not include food?

_____
_____
_____
_____
_____
_____
_____
_____
_____
_____
_____
_____
_____
_____

27. The Power of Our Peers.
Make a list of the people in your life who genuinely support you, and who you can genuinely trust. (Then make time to hang out with them.)

_____
_____
_____
_____
_____
_____
_____
_____
_____
_____
_____
_____
_____
_____
_____
_____

28. Dear Future Me...

Write a letter to your future self to be opened one year from today. What have you accomplished? How do you feel about who you've become? What are your new goals you are working towards?

Ways to stay connected with me.

For more of my grief journey, visit my blog
www.amothersstoryofhealing.wordpress.com

For more health and fitness tips, recipes and workouts visit
www.pammartinfitness.com

For information on my nutrition company and what I recommend go to **www.vibrantfitlife.com**

Find me on social media

 www.facebook.com/pam.martin86

 www.instagram.com/pammartinfitness

Email me at **pam@pammartinfitness.com**

For more information about Fibromuscular Dysplasia visit the Fibromuscular Dysplasia Society of America
http://www.fmdsa.org/fmd_info/what_is_fmd

If "The Girl in the Mirror" helped you, please help me by leaving a 5 star review and your comments on Amazon! That will help me help more people going through their own struggles. God bless you.

Xoxo, Pamela

About the Author:

I am a married mother and grandmother and have had a passion for books for as long as I can remember. My dream of being a published author started in high school when I began writing poetry and short stories. Growing up in rural Missouri on a cattle farm was a great place to feed my imagination and I would write about my experiences.

In 2017, I began putting my journey into words in the hopes that I could help others by sharing my personal story. After talking with so many women who struggle with body image and weight wellness, I felt the pull to reach a broader audience and began writing, *"The Girl in the Mirror"*. Part of my journey includes a tragic loss in my family. My son of 28 years suddenly passed away and I share some of that grief experience in this book as it pertains to my wellness journey. In 2018, I finished my debut book with its release in July. Giving hope to women across the globe who wonder if they can succeed with their goals of a healthy life or withstand the pain tremendous loss brings is my ultimate goal for this book.

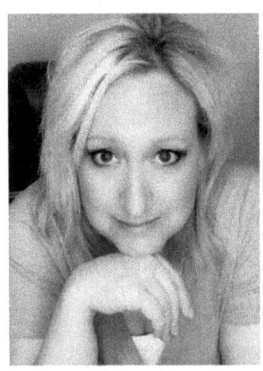

When I am not writing, I am coaching women with fitness and health solutions and loving on my two grandchildren who are the lights of my life. I reside in my hometown in Eastern Missouri with my husband and 3 dogs: Henry, Molly and Leo.

www.ingramcontent.com/pod-product-compliance
Lightning Source LLC
Chambersburg PA
CBHW071316110426
42743CB00042B/2645